Card

MW00324382

A Beginner's Step-by-Step Guide to a Heart-Healthy Life with Recipes and a Meal Plan

Disclaimer

By reading this disclaimer, you are accepting the terms of the disclaimer in full. If you disagree with this disclaimer, please do not read the book. The content in this book is provided for informational and educational purposes only.

This book is not intended to be a substitute for the original work of this diet plan. At most, this book is intended to be a beginner's supplement to the original work for this diet plan and never acts as a direct substitute. This book is an overview, review, and commentary on the facts of that diet plan.

All product names, diet plans, or names used in this book are for identification purposes only and are property of their respective owners. The use of these names does not imply endorsement. All other trademarks cited herein are the property of their respective owners.

None of the information in this book should be accepted as an independent medical or other professional advice.

Table of Contents

Introduction

I want to thank you and congratulate you on getting this guide.

Cardiovascular diseases remain to be one of the leading causes of death worldwide. As such, numerous studies have been conducted over the years to develop effective means of lowering the risk for heart issues and improving the health condition of those who already have heart problems.

One of these methods is through the adaptation of the cardiac diet, which is composed of the following elements:
- Fresh and brightly colored vegetables
- Fresh fruits
- Unrefined, whole grains
- Plant-based food products
- Lean cuts of meat
- Healthy fats
- Anti-inflammatory beverages

Through the cardiac diet, you will be able to normalize your blood pressure, lower down your weight through the reduction of body fat, reduce your glucose levels, and improve the overall performance of your immune system. As confirmed by multiple research studies, the nutritional value of this diet has a greater effect than most cardiovascular medications available today.

In this guide, you will learn how to successfully apply the principles of the cardiac diet in your day-to-day life. Using a sample 7-day meal plan as your starting point, you will learn in later chapters how to sustain your new heart-friendly lifestyle. Once you have working knowledge on what to eat and what to avoid, this book shall also equip you with the proven strategies on how to maximize the effects of the cardiac diet in protecting and promoting the wellness of your heart.

Thanks again for getting this book, I hope you enjoy it!

Chapter 1 – The Heart of the Matter

Given the high prevalence of heart-related health problems, it is a surprise that many people remain uninformed about the forms that it can take, the types of treatments available nowadays, and more importantly, the preventive measures that a person may take. Before delving into the details of the latter, you should first learn what cardiovascular diseases are.

One of the common misconceptions about cardiovascular diseases is that it always involves a heart attack. Because of this, other related health symptoms are either ignored or dismissed until it is already too late for corrective actions to be carried out successfully. Many also assume that it is only linked to high cholesterol levels in the heart. However, studies have shown that cardiovascular diseases are also associated with high blood pressure, insulin resistance, and type-2 diabetes.

Depending on one's lifestyle and genetic makeup, a person may develop any of the following types of cardiovascular diseases:
- Angina
  More commonly known as chest pains, this condition is caused by inadequate blood flow into the muscles of the heart.
- Arteriosclerosis

Also referred to as the coronary-artery disease, this is characterized by the hardening of arteries.

- Atherosclerosis
  When plaques or fatty deposits form, the blood flow to the heart through the arteries becomes clogged up.
- Congestive Heart Failure
  This results from the severe fluid retention within the heart, which happens when the pumping of the heart muscles becomes weakened for a certain period.

The Relationship Between Cardiovascular Diseases and Diet

A landmark study about the risk factors for cardiovascular diseases has revealed that around 90% is within the individual's control. The list includes:

- High levels of bad cholesterol
- Smoking
- Both types of diabetes
- High blood pressure
- Large waistline due to abdominal fat
- High levels of stress
- Low intake of fruits and vegetables
- Sedentary lifestyle

Looking through this list, it is easy to see that one of the first steps that you may take to prevent and combat cardiovascular diseases is improving your diet.

It is important to note that the cardiac diet will not eliminate all of the above-given risk factors. However, the nutrients you can gain from it will strengthen your body well enough to handle the bad effects of stress and smoking.

Chapter 2 – Sample Meal Plan for a Healthier Heart

To get you started, here is a 7-day sample meal plan based on the principles of the cardiac diet, as discussed in further detail in the next chapter. Take note that the recipes for items that have been marked with an asterisk (*) can be found in chapter 7 of this book.

You may also notice later on that each dinner plan involves a glass of red wine. Later on, you will the importance of consuming moderate alcohol in protecting your heart from diseases. If you are abstaining from alcohol, then you may replace this with either tea or plain water.

Day 1
- Breakfast
    - Wholegrain Cereal with Raisins
    - Soymilk

- Morning Snack
    - Banana Slices
    - Plain Water

- Lunch
    - Tomato and Basil Salad
    - Ginger Pumpkin Soup
    - Non-Fat Yoghurt
    - Lemon Water

- Afternoon Snack
    - Dried apricots
    - English Tea

- Dinner
    - Oriental-Style Salmon Fillet
    - Apple and Onion Mix*
    - Dry Red Wine

Day 2
- Breakfast
    - Banana Oatmeal Muffin
    - Green Tea

- Morning Snack
    - Fresh Fruit Cup
    - Plain Water

- Lunch
    - Shrimp & Egg Fried Rice*

- Afternoon Snack
    - Wholegrain Crackers
    - Hummus Dip
    - Water with Cucumber Slices

- Dinner
    - Chicken & Green Beans Stir-Fry
    - Greek Salad
    - Dry Red Wine

Day 3
- Breakfast
  - Toasted Bread with Honey
  - Strawberry Slices
  - Plain Water

- Morning Snack
  - Carrot Sticks
  - Green Smoothie

- Lunch
  - Broccoli Mushroom Bisque
  - Napa Cabbage Salad with Oriental Peanut Dressing
  - Plain Water

- Afternoon Snack
  - Banana Chips
  - Plain Water

- Dinner
  - Grilled Eggplant*
  - Turkey Salad
  - Dry Red Wine

Day 4
- Breakfast
  - Honey-Sweetened Granola Bars
  - English Tea

- Morning Snack
  - Dried Mixed Berries

- o Plain Water

- Lunch
  - o Pepper Ginger Beef Stir-Fry*
  - o Feta Fruit Salad
  - o Plain Water

- Afternoon Snack
  - o Spinach and Kale Smoothie

- Dinner
  - o Mushroom and Kale Casserole
  - o Turkey and Black Bean Burgers
  - o Dry Red Wine

Day 5
- Breakfast
  - o Cherry Oatmeal
  - o Toasted Whole Wheat Bread
  - o Plain Water

- Morning Snack
  - o Apple Slices
  - o Lemon Water

- Lunch
  - o Baked Eggplant Slices
  - o Lettuce, Arugula, White Beans, And Tomato Salad with Italian Dressing
  - o Plain Water

- Afternoon Snack

- o Mixed Berries Smoothie

- Dinner
  - o Salmon & Asparagus*
  - o Dry Red Wine

Day 6
- Breakfast
  - o Chickpea Omelet with Onions and Mushroom
  - o English Tea

- Morning Snack
  - o Banana Bread*
  - o English Tea

- Lunch
  - o Taco Salad Wraps
  - o Butternut Squash & Turmeric Soup*
  - o Plain Water

- Afternoon Snack
  - o Strawberry Slices
  - o Plain Water

- Dinner
  - o Mixed Greens and Orange Salad with Honey-Miso Dressing
  - o Avocado and Cheese Sandwich
  - o Dry Red Wine

Day 7

- Breakfast
    - Dark Chocolate Muffin
    - Ginger Tea

- Morning Snack
    - Blueberry Smoothie

- Lunch
    - Cheddar Turkey Deviled Egg *
    - Steamed Asparagus
    - Lemon Water

- Afternoon Snack
    - Melon Slices
    - Plain Water

- Dinner
    - Broccoli and Chickpea Salad
    - Baked Eggplant and Tomato Slices with Parmesan and Parsley
    - Dry Red Wine

Chapter 3 – Week 1: Understanding the Cardiac Diet Food Pyramid

A comprehensive understanding of the foundations of the cardiac diet is necessary for the successful adaption and sustainability of this diet in your day to day life. Therefore, your first objective is to understand the guiding principles of the cardiac diet in the form of a specialized food pyramid.

In the regular food pyramid, the main sources of protein—meat, poultry, and seafood—are identified as a single food group. The same goes for the primary sources of carbohydrates and fats. Basing your diet in this food pyramid may put you at risk of getting cardiovascular diseases due to the lack of distinction between the good sources and bad sources of macronutrients.

Because of this, the US Department of Food and Agriculture (USDA) has formulated a revised food guide, as illustrated in the food pyramid below:

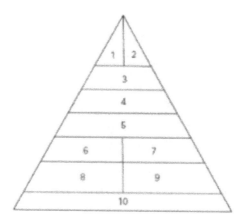

- At the top of this pyramid are:
  - (1) red meats and butter; and
  - (2) pasta, white bread, white rice, potatoes, and sweet treats

  Your daily intake of these food groups should be as minimal as possible.

- The 3rd food group consists of other dairy products and calcium supplements. You must have around 1 to 2 servings of these items per day.

- Next, you must also consume 1 to 2 servings per day of seafood, poultry, and eggs, which make up the 4th food group.

- Nuts and legumes are found in the 5th food group. Try to have at least 3 servings of these food products per day.

- The 6th group is composed of vegetables, which you must consume in great quantities for each meal of the day.

- Rather than sweet desserts, you should eat more fresh fruits instead since they form the 7th food group in this pyramid.

- As the 8th food group, whole grain foods must be incorporate in almost every meal that you will have for each day.

- Plant-based oils, especially extra-virgin olive oil and vegetable oil, should be your primary source of fats every day. These products form the 9th food group in the cardiac diet food pyramid.

- At the base of this food pyramid is a moderately low-calorie diet and weight control.

You might be wondering about the foundation of this new food pyramid. USDA decided to highlight this to show the importance of staying active and keeping a lean body.

Apparently, consuming the right kinds of food is not sufficient in achieving and maintaining a healthy heart. You must also be mindful of your daily caloric intake, and body weight. Even if your current weight belongs to the normal range, a high-calorie diet would still put you at risk of cardiovascular diseases and other serious health conditions.

Now that you have a thorough understanding of the food pyramid for the cardiac diet, your primary focus now lies in the process of integrating it into your life. A study published in the American Psychological Association's Journal by researchers at UCLA has noted that a massive two-thirds of 31 long term studies have had failures in their diet. As stated, one of the primary reasons that people fail in their diets is that it is plain terrible. Diets force people to eat foods that are only found in a brief list of sparsely diverse foods. Another point made by the study is that people who enter a diet start losing weight but fail in the long term. An immediate spike in the loss of weight during a diet can be attributed to the optimism of people trying out a "new thing." But if you do not like the diet, eventually, optimism fades and the resurgence of how awful the diet makes people quit.

To avoid piling up in the statistics, you should arm yourself with knowledge. Starting with the food pyramid, you can pick the foods that you want to eat and the food that you can eat (easily accessible). Following the portions set by the pyramid and eating tasty, readily accessible meals would be a stepping stone into creating a habit.

For a diet to be successful, you need to transform it into a habit. The more a diet is ingrained to oneself, the more it is easier to do and the less our body will reject it. Start the week by compiling a list of the food that you can take in. Take note of the quantities that are healthy for you according to the pyramid.

Another point to consider is to start gradually. Introduce healthier and healthier foods into your meals as the days go by. If you encounter a certain food that might not be appetizing for you, try to experiment with it using the foods that you already like.

It may also be helpful that you keep track of your progress within the week. Use a notebook to record your progress. During challenging times, the records of your progress will be a breathing space of sorts. It will show you what you have already done and what you can further do. Keeping records not only clears your path to your goal but it could also be a way to praise yourself for your achievements.

People hate change, that is why entering into a new diet is exceedingly difficult. But if you make that change gradual, it will be easier to adopt. If you make it interesting, fun and give a sense of achievement, it will form a habit.

Chapter 4 – Week 2: Identifying the Good Fats vs. Bad Fats

As explained during the previous chapter, one of the critical lessons that you need to learn when adapting the cardiac diet is how to distinguish the sources of good fats from the bad ones. Though it may sound counterintuitive for most beginners, the right kind of fats can be beneficial for the heart. They are essential in raising the levels of good cholesterol, which in turn is important in the generation of energy within the body.

To figure out where you may obtain good fats, you must first learn the forms that they can take. In the cardiac diet, there are two kind of good fats:

- Monounsaturated fats
  Primary Contribution: lowers the level of bad cholesterol; lowers the risk of insulin resistance
  Sources: olive oil, avocado oil, peanut oil, flaxseed, canola oil

- Omega-3 fatty acids
  Primary Contribution: increases the level of good cholesterol; improves the elasticity of the artery walls

Sources: walnuts, flaxseeds, soybeans, canola oil, salmon, albacore tuna

On the other hand, bad fats are harmful to the body since they will increase one's risk of getting various forms of cardiovascular diseases. Though they should be avoided at all costs, bad fats are more widely used and more readily available than the good fats, mainly due to their lower cost, higher supply, and generally longer shelf-life.

As such, it is important for you to always be wary of the products that you are going to buy and consume. To help you through this, here are the types of bad fats to avoid, and their respective sources:

- Saturated fats
  Primary Contribution: increases the production of cholesterol, which can then lead to blood clotting; prolonged overconsumption of these fats can significantly increase the risk of heart attack and stroke.
  Sources: full-fat dairy products, fatty cuts of meat, margarine, coconut oil

- Trans fat
  Primary Contribution: increases the level of bad cholesterol; lowers the level of good cholesterol, increases inflammation in the blood vessels; increases the level of triglycerides, which then increase the likelihood of blood clot formation.
  Sources: corn oil, margarine, liquid shortening, fast food products

Now that you have identified the possible sources of good fats and bad fats, you must now try to incorporate them into your daily diet. Remember, balance is key.

Here are some tips to get you started on this:

- Use cold-water varieties of fish, such as albacore tuna, mackerel, and salmon, for at least 4 to 6 dishes in your weekly meal plan.
- Make extra-virgin olive oil your primary cooking oil and dressing. You may also use this as a replacement for your butter spread or as the base of your pasta sauce.
- Sprinkle chopped nuts or lightly toasted seeds as toppings for your salad.
- Skim off the fat that will form on top of the soup, stew, or whatever dish that contains animal fat.
- Always read the labels of dairy products before buying them. Remember, skimmed milk contains no fat at all. Yogurt is another heart-friendly dairy product, with only 15% fat-from-calories content.

Nobody likes a rupturing plaque in their arteries. You do not need to be a doctor to know that a rupturing plaque in the heart is – catastrophic. While a plaque in the artery is still a terrible thing, the verdict on the health effects of fat is now being questioned. Since the 1960s we were all lead to believe that dietary fat is the highest of all evils and is the worst thing that we can put in our mouth.

But recent investigations conducted by Columbia University's Mailman School of Public Health and the City University of New York has unearthed evidence that we were led to believe a half false statement. It is a shocker for many people to know that fats are good for you (well, not every type of fat).

Since the 1960s we have steadily removed fat from our diets citing its "health risk," that is why it could be no surprise that a lot of people are averse to eating anything with a fat level greater than zero stamped onto it. Even knowing that there are good and bad types of fats will prevent a lot of people from eating good fat. People might say that it is a much safer bet to eat not fat at all. But fat is integral to our body's nutritional needs.

Week Two should be focused on introducing yourself to good fats. As mentioned previously, you must have by now the ability to choose foods that are rich in good fats. Make week two as a starting ground for choosing the right type of food that will give you the maximum amount of good fats that you need.

Just like week one, start introducing yourself to the diets that are rich in good fats. Pick out the foods that you like or are already eating and start integrating them into your meals. It does not need to be the main dish.

By this week, you can start narrowing down the food types which you are comfortable with. Narrowing down your food list does not mean that it is all you will ever eat throughout the diet. But having a set of food items that you are comfortable with lets you ease your way into the cardiac diet.

When you have already made a habit of following the cardiac diet, you can expand to newer foods. You could make your meals interesting by adding new food on the dining table each week onwards.

It might be baby steps, but baby steps came before we can walk. And walking came before we can run.

Chapter 5 - Week 3: Heart-Friendly Food Handling Techniques

Through the right preparation and cooking techniques, you will be able to reduce the number of calories in your food, as well as eliminate the usage of trans fat and saturated fats.

Your goal for the third week of your cardiac diet is to prepare and cook your food following the techniques specified below.

Using the knowledge you have gained in the previous chapters, you may now try creating your own cardiac diet meal plan. In case you are not quite sure which dishes to include in your plan, feel free to reuse your favorite meals from the sample weekly plan.

Preparation Techniques
- Before cooking poultry, pork, beef, and other meat products, remove the skin, and cut off all visible fats.
  - However, do not remove the skin if you are going to roast it. This will prevent the meat from drying out. Instead, discard the skin after you have roasted it.

- When baking, wrap your food in cooking parchment. This will allow you to retain the natural of juices within the food.
- To produce the same effect when grilling, wrap your food in aluminum foil.
- Wrapping the food for steaming in either cabbage leaves or lettuce will help you keep the moisture inside the filling.

Cooking Techniques
- Steaming

  Choose this method if you want the natural flavor and color of the food to be maintained after cooking. Many heart-conscious people prefer steaming their food because there is less nutrient loss during the process. You also do not need to add fat to cook the food.

  Steaming works well not just vegetables, but also for poultry products. In case you to enhance the flavor of your steamed food, you may throw in some herbs into the water that you will use during steaming.

  Just be sure that the level of water below will not reach the food you are steaming. Otherwise, you will end up boiling your food.

- Stir-Frying

This is a relatively quick method that utilizes very high temperatures. Therefore, you should complete your preparations first before starting this process. Use a large skillet or wok for the best results.

- Roasting
  You can roast your food without having to add oils and fat. Though you may be tempted to let your food sit in its fat drippings to let the flavor back in, the cardiac diet discourages this practice.

Special Tips on Handling Meats, Poultry, and Seafood

- Always remove any solidified fats that will form on top of your soups, stews, and sauces that uses meats or poultry products as their ingredients.
- If you want to reuse the marinade you have used for your meats, poultry, or seafood, make sure to boil the marinade for around 5 minutes first. After then, you are free to use the marinade for your sauces, or for basting the meats, poultry, seafood you are cooking.
- Rather than frying fish, opt to either bake or grill the fish instead, along with fresh herbs and citrus slices.

Special Tips on Handling Vegetables

- Avoid overcooking vegetables. They will not only lose their taste but will also lose the vitamins and minerals they contain. Aim for a tender-crisp texture the next time you cook vegetables.
- You can lessen the percentage of meats or poultry in your casseroles, stews, and soups by increasing the number of vegetables in the recipe. To prevent any significant change in appearance, you may finely chop your vegetables and herbs.

The Japanese call it Fugu – one of the deadliest fish in the sea, also one of the most delectable. If you catch a Fugu, fried it, and ate it, you would not be here reading this. But by carefully preparing the Fugu, the Japanese have made it safe for consumption. The careful preparation made eating the savory Fugu possible.

Using Fugu as an example, we can view the trans fats and unhealthy aspects of our food as the toxin. Unhealthy eating would not kill you within seconds but eventually, it will kill you. But just like the Fugu, we can learn techniques to carefully prepare our food for consumption. By properly preparing them, we can remove most if not all the unhealthy fats and excess calories in our food. We can even make healthy food healthier through careful preparation.

For the past two weeks, you may already have built a list of food that you like to eat, that is enjoyable, and that is accessible. You may have already eliminated as well those that are a major source of bad fats.

Using the techniques mentioned in this chapter, make your list healthier and much more In line with the cardiac diet. The techniques mentioned are not just for your list, you can also use it to explore other food groups or alternatives. An example could be poultry, you might not have included it into your list by week two seeing that it could lead to a problem and detract you from the cardio diet. You can challenge yourself by exploring food groups such as poultry and making it healthier for your consumption.

You are encouraged to explore as much as you like with the food groups and experiment on which one you like. The important thing is that by this week, you should already have a rough sketch of the type of meals that you can sustain, enjoy, and afford. By far the types of food you will be choosing this week for your cardiac diet is going to be your plan for a couple of months that you will be taking baby steps. Once you are accustomed to it, you will begin making more meals that are fun and heart-healthy.

Throughout the cardiac diet, challenge yourself by making it enjoyable. Do not forget to continue recording your steps and make each meal an achievement and a celebration.

This will be the last chapter talking about food consumption. In the next chapter, we will be talking about a major topic in diet plans – and it is more than just water.

Chapter 6 – Week 4: Supplementing Your Cardiac Diet Meal Plan with Anti-Inflammatory Beverages

Unlike other healthy diets that prohibit the consumption of alcohol, the cardiac diet allows its followers to consume moderate amounts of wine, particularly dry red wine.

This principle is based on a study conducted among the French, who have a low heart disease-related mortality rate, despite having a diet that consists mostly of saturated fats.

Researchers have discovered that it is a red wine that possesses antioxidant properties that can counterbalance the supposed negative effects of their diet. As such, they have dubbed this observation as the "French paradox".

The key to properly implementing this as part of your cardiac diet is moderation. Experts recommend a maximum of one glass of red wine per day among women, while men can have a maximum of two glasses per day.

When consumed in moderation, you will be able to unlock the following benefits of red wine to your health:
- Lowered risk of heart diseases.
- Lowered risk of type-2 diabetes; and

- Fewer cases of inflammation across different parts of your body.

Since grape seeds and grape skin contain the highest levels of polyphenols—or antioxidant compounds, you should opt for red wines made of organically grown grapes.

You should also get wines produced in climates that are cool and damp to ensure that you will be getting more resveratrol, which is one of the most potent forms of polyphenol. In case you are not sure which kind of red wine fits these criteria, it has been reported that Shiraz and Pinot Noir contain lots of resveratrol compared to other popular varieties of wine.

Alternative Anti-Inflammatory Beverages
In case that you do not or cannot drink alcohol—whether by choice, or a result of your current condition, such as pregnancy—you may opt to drink tea instead.

According to studies, white, green, and black tea all contain varying amounts of antioxidant catechins. The fewer process the tea has gone through, the more catechins it will retain. Therefore, to maximize the antioxidants you may get from your cup of tea, you should go for either white tea or green tea.

Aside from benefiting from its anti-inflammatory properties, tea can also help in maintaining your weight within the ideal range. Many people have also reported being more energized due to the regular consumption of tea.

The recommended amount of catechins per day is 300 mg for normal-sized adults. This should be equivalent to around 2 to 3 cups of tea per day, depending on the brand.

This chapter goes to show that a good and healthy diet does not have to be an arduous one. For most diets, the main philosophy is to furlough most beverages. Often, diets recommend one drink only –water. While drinking solely water is beneficial and does not have a downside, it may affect your entire experience of the diet. Most diets seem to look at beverages other than water as bad, which is not true. By discouraging beverages other than water, a great amount of healthy nutrition is being missed by a lot of people.

For three weeks you have been learning the proper types of food to eat, the truth about fats, and how you can prepare and customize your meals for a healthier and enjoyable experience.

One of the key reasons why obesity is rampant is due to what we call "liquid calories." These calories come from beverages that we drink. The reason they are unhealthy is that they are filled to the brim with additives to make them "taste good." Being a liquid, you can drink a lot of these beverages without being full. The feeling of fullness is what limits our body's caloric intake. Liquid calories override that important function for our bodies.

While the cardiac diet allows for beverages with beneficial effects, it is by far not a free for all. It is strongly recommended that a sense of "moderation" is always put to mind. Since our bodies can be overridden by the so-called "liquid calories" it is important for us to police ourselves.

Always make a mental note of your consumption of these beverages whether alcoholic or not. In moderation, these beverages far out-weighs it is any added calories. But at a much larger consumption, it will prove to have negative impacts.

Learn moderation and hopefully, it can help you moderate your meals as well. Keep a mental note or better yet record each consumption. AS with the previous chapter, make a consumption, therefore the cardiac diet, enjoyable and interesting.

Chapter 7- Recipe List

Refer to the recipes below for suggested dishes that best exemplifies the principles of the cardiac diet. Each has been carefully incorporated into the meal plan given earlier to give a background on the makings an ideal heart-friendly meal plan.

If you want to substitute any of the ingredients below, or if you think that there is a better way of cooking these dishes, then feel free to experiment, as long as you will remain within the confines of what is allowable in the cardiac diet. When in doubt, refer back to the cardiac diet food pyramid, and the various tips and suggestions given in the preceding chapters.

- Apple and Onion Mix

  Ingredients:
  - ✓ 1 medium-sized Granny Smith apple, finely diced
  - ✓ ¼ cup red onion, finely chopped
  - ✓ ¼ cup walnuts, toasted, finely chopped
  - ✓ 1 tablespoon extra-virgin olive oil OR walnut oil
  - ✓ 1 teaspoon lemon juice

- ✓ 1 teaspoon honey
- ✓ ½ teaspoon sage, finely chopped
- ✓ A pinch of salt

Procedure:

1. Place apple dices, chopped onion, chopped walnuts, chopped sage, oil, honey, and lemon juice in a bowl.
2. Toss until all ingredients are evenly distributed and coated with honey-lemon dressing.
3. Sprinkle with salt to taste.
4. Serve immediately.

Yield: 1 to 2 servings

- Shrimp and Egg Fried Rice

  Ingredients:

  - ✓ ¾ cup long-grained jasmine rice washed
  - ✓ ½ cup of water
  - ✓ 1 cup chicken broth, no salt
  - ✓ 4 ounces large shrimps (around 35 pieces per pound), peeled and deveined, sliced into ½-inch bits, patted dry
  - ✓ 2 large eggs, beaten

- ✓ 2 cups sugar snap peas, trimmed and cut into two
- ✓ 1 cup shiitake mushrooms, caps only
- ✓ 1 cup carrots, diced into 1/4-inch bits
- ✓ 2 tablespoons low-sodium soy sauce
- ✓ 1 tablespoon garlic, minced
- ✓ 1 tablespoon fresh ginger, minced
- ✓ ¼ teaspoon red chili pepper, crushed
- ✓ 2 tablespoons vegetable oil
- ✓ 1/8 teaspoon ground white pepper

Procedure:

1. Combine and boil the chicken broth and water into a small saucepan.
2. Add washed jasmine rice.
3. Reduce the heat to low.
4. Cover the saucepan with its lid.
5. Simmer until the rice has become tender, and the liquid has vaporized.
6. Remove from heat.
7. In a frying pan, heat the vegetable oil for half a minute.

8. Add minced garlic, minced ginger, and crushed red chili peppers.

9. Stir fry using a metal spatula for about 10 seconds, or until mixture has become fragrant.

10. Add diced carrots and mushroom caps.

11. Stir fry for about 1 minute.

12. Add shrimp slices.

13. Stir fry for another minute.

14. Add sugar snap pear halves.

15. Stir fry for 1 minute, or until peas have turned bright green.

16. Remove from heat.

17. Add beaten eggs, cooked rice, soy sauce, and pepper.

18. While still off the heat, stir fry for about 1 to minutes, or until shrimp are cooked through and the eggs have set.

19. Transfer into a bowl and serve while it is still hot.

Yield: 2 to 3 servings

- Grilled Eggplant

Ingredients:

- ✓ 2 small eggplants OR 1 large eggplant (around 1 ¼ to 1 ½ pound in total), sliced into ½-inch thick rounds

- ✓ 2 tablespoons extra-virgin olive oil

- ✓ A pinch of salt

Procedure:

1. Pre-heat the grill using the medium-high setting.

2. Toss eggplant slices and olive oil in a bowl.

3. Sprinkle with salt to taste.

4. Toss the ingredients again.

5. Place eggplant slices into the grill.

6. Turn over to the other side after about 4 minutes, or until charred spots have appeared on the underside.

7. Continue grilling until eggplant slices have become tender.

Yield: 2 servings

Tip: You can prepare this dish ahead of time. Just place into an airtight container once it has cooled down, and then refrigerate. Grilled eggplant can last for up to 4 days in chilled condition.

- Mixed Vegetable Roast with Lemon Zest

Ingredients:

- ✓ 1½ cups broccoli florets
- ✓ 1½ cups cauliflower florets
- ✓ ¾ cup red bell pepper, diced by 1-inch cuts
- ✓ ¾ cup zucchini, diced by 1-inch cuts
- ✓ 2 thinly sliced cloves of garlic
- ✓ lemon zest (2 teaspoons)
- ✓ olive oil (1 tablespoon)
- ✓ ¼ teaspoon salt
- ✓ 1 teaspoon dried and crushed oregano

Procedure:

1. Preheat oven set to 425°F.

2. Combine garlic and both florets (broccoli and cauliflower) in a baking pan (15-by-10-inch). Drizzle oil over the vegetables and sprinkle with salt

and oregano; stir long enough to coat. Roast for 10 minutes.

3. Add zucchini and bell pepper to the rest of the mix in the pan; toss to combine. Continue roasting for 10 to 15 minutes more until the pieces are lightly browned and are crisp-tender.

4. Before serving, drizzle lemon zest over the vegetables and toss.

Yield: 1 to 2 servings

- Pepper Ginger Beef Stir-Fry

  Ingredients:

  - ✓ 6 ounces (175 grams) lean rump OR fillet steak, thinly cut into strips across the grain

  - ✓ 2 ounces (55 grams) mange tout, trimmed

  - ✓ 4 spring onions, chopped

  - ✓ 1 small red bell pepper, deseeded and thinly cut into strips

  - ✓ 1 small green OR yellow bell pepper, deseeded and thinly cut into strips

  - ✓ 1 ½ teaspoon Sichuan pepper, crushed

  - ✓ 1 fresh red chili, deseeded and finely chopped

  - ✓ 1 carrot, cut into thin sticks

  - ✓ 0.8-inch (2-cm) fresh ginger, peeled and thinly cut into strips

  - ✓ 1 clove garlic, finely chopped

- ✓ 1 tablespoon low-sodium soy sauce
- ✓ 4 tablespoons water
- ✓ 2-3 teaspoons sunflower oil
- ✓ 1 teaspoon cornflour
- ✓ 1 teaspoon soft dark brown sugar

Procedure:

1. Mix cornflour and water in a small bowl until the texture has become smooth.

2. Stir in soy sauce and sugar until the particles have been completely dissolved. Set aside.

3. In a non-stick wok, heat 1 teaspoon of sunflower oil using the medium setting of the stove.

4. Add the beef strips and crushed pepper.

5. Stir-fry for about 3 to 4 minutes, or until the beef strips have turned brown.

6. Transfer the beef strips into a plate using a slotted spoon. Set aside.

7. Pour the remaining sunflower oil into the work.

8. Heat the oil using the medium setting.

9. Add the garlic, red chili, mange tout, peppers, carrot, spring onions, and ginger into the wok.

10. Stir-fry for 3 to 5 minutes or until preferred texture is achieved.

11. Return the stir-fried beef strips from earlier.

12. Pour the cornflour mixture into the can

13. Stir fry for 1 to minutes, or until beef strips have become hot again.

14. Serve immediately over cooked rice or rice noodles.

Yield: 2 to 3 servings

Tip: If you are allergic to gluten, feel free to replace low-sodium soy sauce used in this recipe with any gluten-free alternative.

- Salmon and Asparagus

  Ingredients:

  ✓ 2 salmon fillets, around 5 ounces (140 grams) each

- ✓ 14 ounces (397 grams) young potatoes

- ✓ 8 asparagus spears, trimmed and halved

- ✓ 2 handfuls cherry tomatoes

- ✓ 1 handful basil leaves

- ✓ 2 tablespoons extra-virgin olive oil

- ✓ 1 tablespoon balsamic vinegar

Procedure:

1. Heat oven to 428 ºF (220 ºC or gas 7 oven fan setting)

2. Arrange the potatoes into a baking dish.

3. Drizzle potatoes with 1 tablespoon extra-virgin olive oil.

4. Roast potatoes for 20 minutes, or until they have turned golden brown.

5. Place the asparagus into the baking dish together with the potatoes.

6. Roast in the oven for another 15 minutes.

7. Arrange the cherry tomatoes and salmon among the vegetables.

8. Drizzle with balsamic vinegar and the remaining olive oil.

9. Roast for 10 to 15 minutes, or until salmon is cooked.

10. Throw in a handful of basil leaves before transferring everything in a serving dish.

11. Serve while hot.

Yield: 2 servings

- Banana Bread

Ingredients:

- ✓ 10.6 ounces (300 grams) overripe bananas, mashed
- ✓ 5 ounces (140 grams) whole-wheat flour
- ✓ 3.5 ounces (100 grams) self-rising flour
- ✓ 3 large eggs, beaten
- ✓ 10 tablespoons natural, low-fat yogurt
- ✓ 4 tablespoons agave syrup
- ✓ 1 teaspoon sodium bicarbonate
- ✓ 1 teaspoon baking powder
- ✓ 0.88-ounce (25 grams) pecan OR walnuts, chopped (optional)
- ✓ low-fat butter spread (for greasing the loaf tin)

Procedure:

1. Heat the oven to 320 °F (160 °C or gas 3 settings).

2. Grease a 2-pound loaf tin before lining it with baking parchment that is at least 1 inch over the top edges.

3. Mix the whole-wheat flour, self-rising flour, sodium bicarbonate, baking powder, and a pinch of salt in a large bowl.

4. Mix the bananas, agave syrup, eggs, and yogurt in a separate bowl.

5. Quickly stir in the wet ingredients into dry ingredients.

6. Gently scrape the batter into the tin.

7. Scatter with chopped nuts on top, if you are using them.

8. Bake for 1 hour-10 min up to 1 hour-15 min, or until a cake tester or skewer comes out clean.

9. Cooldown the bread while it is still in the tin on a wire rack.

10. Serve warm or at ambient temperature, with low-fat spread on the side.

Yield: 6 to 8 servings

- Butternut Squash and Turmeric Soup

  Ingredients:

  - ✓ 1 medium butternut squash (about 2 ½ lbs.), peeled and chopped into 1-inch pieces, reserve the seeds

  - ✓ 2 medium carrots, cut into 1-inch pieces

  - ✓ 2 ¼ teaspoon turmeric powder

  - ✓ 1 large onion, roughly chopped

  - ✓ 2 tablespoons light coconut milk

  - ✓ 1 tablespoon vegetable soup base OR 1 vegetable bouillon cube

  - ✓ 2 ½ tablespoons extra-virgin olive oil

  - ✓ 2 ¼ teaspoon ground black pepper

  Procedure:

  1. Heat 2 tablespoons of oil in a large Dutch oven (cast-iron pot) using medium heat.

2. Add the onion and cover the pot with its lid.

3. Cook, while stirring occasionally, for 6 to 8 minutes, or until onions have become tender.

4. Mix the soup base or bouillon with 6 cups of boiling water.

5. Stir until all powder or cube has been dissolved.

6. Add the carrots, squash, 2 teaspoons of turmeric, and ½ teaspoon of ground black pepper into the pot.

7. Cook for 1 minute while stirring occasionally.

8. Pour the soup broth into the pot.

9. Bring to a boil before reducing the heat.

10. Simmer for 18 to 22 minutes, or until vegetables have become very tender.

11. Heat oven to 375°F (191 ºC).

12. Toss ¼ cup of the reserved seeds with the remaining oil, ¼ teaspoon turmeric, and ¼ teaspoon black pepper.

13. Roast for about 9 to 11 minutes, or until seeds have become crispy and golden brown

14. Puree the soup using an immersion blender.

15. Sprinkle with toasted seeds on top, and swirl in the coconut milk.

16. Serve immediately.

Yield: 3 to 4 servings

Tip: If you do not have an immersion blender, you may opt for a regular blender instead. Just remember to divide the soup into batches to get the right texture.

- Cheddar Turkey Deviled Egg

Ingredients:

- ✓ 6 large organic eggs
- ✓ 2 slices nitrate-free turkey bacon
- ✓ ¼ cup low-fat cheddar cheese, shredded OR grated
- ✓ 3 tablespoons light mayonnaise
- ✓ 1 teaspoon white wine vinegar
- ✓ ½ teaspoon chives, chopped
- ✓ 1/8 teaspoon ground black pepper
- ✓ 1/8 teaspoon salt

Procedure:

1. Place the eggs in a large pot or saucepan.

2. Pour cold water into the pot or pan until the water is covering the eggs by 1 ½ inches.

3. Bring the water to a boil over high heat.

4. Once it has boiled, remove the pot, or pan from the stove.

5. Cover the pot or pan, and let it stand for 12 to 15 minutes.

6. When it has cooled down, peel off the egg's shells.

7. Fry the bacon slices using medium-high heat in a non-stick skillet until bacon slices have become crispy but not burnt.

8. Transfer fried bacon into paper towels to drain off the excess oil.

9. Once it has cooled down, break down the bacon into small bits. Set aside.

10. Cut the hard-boiled eggs into half, lengthwise.

11. Gently carve out the egg yolks into a medium-sized bowl.

12. Arrange the hollowed-out egg halves in a flat container.

13. Add the rest of the ingredients into the bowl with the yolk.

14. Stir well until the texture has become smooth.

15. Transfer the mixture into a piping bag or resealable bag with a trimmed corner.

16. Pipe the yolk mixture back into the egg halves.

17. Sprinkle each filled egg halves with bacon bits.

18. Serve immediately or after it has been chilled for at least half an hour.

Yield: 3 to 4 servings

- Go Green Blueberries

Ingredients:
- ✓ 2 cups chopped spinach
- ✓ 1/4 cup water
- ✓ 1/3 cup chopped carrot
- ✓ 1/2 cup blueberries
- ✓ 1/2 cup chopped cucumber
- ✓ 1/4 cup almond milk
- ✓ 4 ice cubes

Procedure:
1. Using a blender, mix the water and spinach. Slowly turn up the speed until no solid particles are present.
2. After the mixture has homogenized, add the other ingredients.
3. Continue to increase speed until you reach the maximum speed for 30 seconds.
4. Serve chilled.

Yield: 2

- Papa-yum!

Ingredients:
- ✓ 1 cup spinach
- ✓ 1 cup chopped kale
- ✓ 3/4 cup water

- ✓ 1/2 cup chopped cucumber
- ✓ 1 green apple
- ✓ 1 cup chopped papaya
- ✓ 1 tablespoon ground flaxseed

Procedure:

1. Using a blender, mix the water, spinach, and kale. Increase speed until all solid particles are gone.
2. Add the rest of the ingredients. Resume blending until reaching the maximum speed.
3. Maintain the maximum speed for 30 seconds before serving.
4. Serve chilled.

Yield: 2

- Energy Boost Smoothie

Ingredients:
- ✓ 1 large rib celery
- ✓ 1 tablespoon parsley
- ✓ 3/4 cup water
- ✓ 1/2 cup chopped cooked beets
- ✓ 1 small orange, segmented
- ✓ 3/4 cup chopped carrot

Procedure:
1. Using a blender, mix the water, parsley, and celery. Increase speed until all solid particles are gone.
2. Add the rest of the ingredients. Resume blending until reaching the maximum speed.
3. Maintain the maximum speed for 30 seconds before serving.
4. Serve chilled.

Yield: 2

- Anti-Diabetic Smoothie

Ingredients:
- ✓ 2 cups spinach
- ✓ 2 large kale leaves
- ✓ 3/4 cup water
- ✓ 1 large frozen banana
- ✓ 1/2 cup frozen mango

- ✓ 1/2 cup frozen peach
- ✓ 1 tablespoon ground flaxseeds
- ✓ 1 tablespoon almond butter or peanut butter

Procedure:

1. Using a blender, mix the water, spinach, and kale. Increase speed until all solid particles are gone.
2. Add the rest of the ingredients. Resume blending until reaching the maximum speed.
3. Maintain the maximum speed for 30 seconds before serving.
4. Serve chilled.

Yield: 2

- Almond Surf Smoothie

Ingredients:
- ✓ 1 large banana
- ✓ 1 cup almond milk
- ✓ 1 tablespoon almond butter
- ✓ 1 tablespoon wheat germ
- ✓ 1/8 teaspoon vanilla extract
- ✓ 1/8 teaspoon ground cinnamon
- ✓ 3–4 ice cubes

Procedure:
1. Using a blender, place all the ingredients and start blending.
2. Increase speed until you reach the intermediate speed setting.
3. Maintain speed for 30 seconds before serving.
4. Serve chilled.

Yield: 1

- Toasted Almond Banana Mix

Ingredients:
- ✓ 2 slices whole-wheat bread
- ✓ 2 tablespoons almond butter
- ✓ 1 small banana
- ✓ 1/8 teaspoon ground cinnamon

Procedure:

1. Start by toasting each piece of bread.
2. After toasting, add the butter.
3. Add the banana slices and a pinch of cinnamon.
4. Serve Immediately.

Yield: 1

- Berry Blast English Muffin

Ingredients:
- ✓ 1 English muffin, halved
- ✓ 1 tablespoon cream cheese
- ✓ 4 strawberries
- ✓ 1/2 cup blueberries

Procedure:
1. Start by toasting each half of the muffin.
2. After being toasted, add the cream cheese on each half.
3. Add the berries.
4. Serve immediately.

Yield: 1

- Berry Blast Oats

Ingredients:
- ✓ 1 1/2 cups plain almond milk
- ✓ 1/8 teaspoon vanilla extract
- ✓ 1 cup oats
- ✓ 3/4 cup mix of blueberries and blackberries
- ✓ 2 tablespoons toasted pecans

Procedure:
1. With a small frying pan, warm up the vanilla and almond milk together using medium fire.
2. Right before the ingredients boil, add the oat. Cook for 5 minutes.
3. Add the berries.
4. Serve hot.

Yield: 2

- Apple Cinnamon Smash Oatmeal

Ingredients:
- ✓ 1 1/2 cups plain almond milk
- ✓ 1 cup oats
- ✓ 1 large Granny Smith apple
- ✓ 1/4 teaspoon ground cinnamon
- ✓ 2 tablespoons toasted walnut pieces

Procedure:

1. Heat the apple and oats together in low to medium fire.
2. Continue heating for 5 minutes.
3. Add the cinnamon.
4. Serve hot.

Yield: 2

- Energizing Oatmeal

Ingredients:

- ✓ 1/4 cup water
- ✓ 1/4 cup milk
- ✓ 1/2 cup oats
- ✓ 4 egg whites
- ✓ 1/8 teaspoon ground cinnamon
- ✓ 1/8 teaspoon ground ginger
- ✓ 1/4 cup blueberries

Procedure:

1. Start by mixing the milk and water in a pan.
2. Heat the mixture on the stove using medium settings.
3. Just before the mixture boils, add the oats and continue heating for 5 minutes.
4. Mix in the whites, continue cooking for 4 minutes.
5. Add the ginger and cinnamon.
6. Serve hot.

Yield: 1

- Quinoa-based Oriental Salad

Ingredients:
- ✓ 2 cups uncooked quinoa
- ✓ 4 cups vegetable broth
- ✓ 1 cup edamame
- ✓ 1/4 cup chopped green onion
- ✓ 1 1/2 teaspoons chopped fresh mint
- ✓ 1/2 cup chopped carrot
- ✓ 1/2 cup chopped red bell pepper
- ✓ 1/8 teaspoon pepper flakes
- ✓ 1/2 teaspoon grated orange zest
- ✓ 2 tablespoons chopped fresh Thai basil
- ✓ Juice from half an orange
- ✓ 1 teaspoon sesame seeds
- ✓ 1 tablespoon sesame oil
- ✓ 1 tablespoon olive oil
- ✓ 1/8 teaspoon black pepper

Procedure:
1. Mix the broth and quinoa in a pan.
2. Set the stove to high and place the pan. Let the mixture heat up for 12 to 14 minutes.
3. After heating, cover the pan and wait for 4 minutes.
4. Place the mixture in a separate container and add the rest of the ingredients.
5. Let it cool down before serving.

Yield: 6

- Hearty Chicken Salad with Pasta

Ingredients:
- ✓ 8 ounces penne pasta
- ✓ 1 (6-ounce) chicken breast
- ✓ 1 cup seedless red grapes
- ✓ 1/4 cup walnut pieces
- ✓ 1 tablespoon red wine vinegar
- ✓ 1/2 cup chopped celery
- ✓ 1/2 cup Greek yogurt
- ✓ 1/2 teaspoon black pepper
- ✓ 1/8 teaspoon salt

Procedure:
1. Start by cooking the pasta, a small addition of cooking oil is recommended.
2. Continue cooking the pasta for 7 – 9 minutes before removing the water.
3. Remove the fat off the chicken and chop it into small pieces.
4. Boil some water and place the chopped chicken into it. Boil for 7 minutes.
5. Remove water from both ingredients.
6. Add both the chicken and pasta together with the rest of the ingredients.
7. Cooldown before serving.

Yield: 6

- Heart Helping Cobb

Ingredients:
- ✓ 4 slices turkey bacon
- ✓ 5 cups spinach
- ✓ 1 cup sliced cremini mushrooms
- ✓ 1/2 cup shredded carrot
- ✓ 1/2 cucumber
- ✓ 1/2 (15-ounce) can kidney beans
- ✓ 1 large avocado
- ✓ 1/3 cup crumbled blue cheese

Procedure:
1. Coat your frying pan with oil.
2. Place the bacon and turkey. Cook for 7 minutes.
3. Cut both bacon and turkey into small pieces.
4. Arrange on the plate with the rest of the ingredients.
5. Serve hot.

Yield: 4

- Grenade Salad

Ingredients:
- ✓ 4 cups arugula
- ✓ 1 large avocado
- ✓ 1/2 cup sliced fennel
- ✓ 1/2 cup sliced Anjou pears
- ✓ 1/4 cup pomegranate seeds

Procedure:
1. Add together all the ingredients aside from the pomegranate seeds.
2. After mixing well, add the seeds and mix well.
3. Serve with any type of desired dressing.

Yield: 4

- Chicken Breast Delight

Ingredients:
- ✓ 1 teaspoon dried oregano
- ✓ 1/2 teaspoon rosemary
- ✓ 1/2 teaspoon garlic powder
- ✓ 1/8 teaspoon salt
- ✓ Finely ground Black pepper
- ✓ 4 chicken breasts

Procedure:
1. Remove any fat from the breasts.
2. Mix the remaining ingredients in a separate container.
3. Add the mixture on either side of the chicken.
4. Prepare a frying pan, lightly oil the pan, and set the stove to medium.
5. Add the chicken into the frying pan. Cook for 3 to 5 minutes on each face.
6. Cool the chicken for a couple of minutes after cooking.
7. Serve warm.

Yield: 4

- Sun Crust Turkey Cuts

Ingredients:
- ✓ 2 (6-ounce) turkey breasts
- ✓ 1 1/2 cups sunflower seeds
- ✓ 1/4 teaspoon ground cumin
- ✓ 2 tablespoons chopped parsley
- ✓ 1/4 teaspoon paprika
- ✓ 1/4 teaspoon cayenne pepper
- ✓ 1/4 teaspoon black pepper
- ✓ 1/3 cup whole wheat flour
- ✓ 3 egg whites

Procedure:
1. Start by warming up the oven to around 395 degrees F.
2. Prepare the breasts by cutting it into ¼ inch thick slices.
3. Mix the parsley, paprika, cumin, cayenne, sunflower seeds, and pepper in a processor.
4. Prepare the whites and flour in a separate container each.
5. Coat each breast part with the mixtures separately starting with the flour mixture, proceeding to the whites and then the processed mixture.
6. After coating all breasts, prepare the pan.
7. Bake the breasts for approximately 12 minutes on the oven.

8. Flip each side and resume baking for another 12 minutes.
9. Serve hot.

Yield: 4

- Turkish Meatballs in Marinara

Ingredients:
- ✓ 1-pound ground turkey
- ✓ 1/2 small onion
- ✓ 2 large cloves garlic,
- ✓ 1/4 cup red bell pepper
- ✓ 3 tablespoons chopped parsley
- ✓ 1/2 teaspoon pepper flakes
- ✓ 1/8 teaspoon ground cumin
- ✓ 1/2 teaspoon dried Pre-mixed Italian herbs
- ✓ 1/8 teaspoon black pepper
- ✓ 1 egg
- ✓ 1/4 cup breadcrumbs
- ✓ 1/8 teaspoon salt
- ✓ 4 tablespoons olive oil
- ✓ 1 (16-ounce) jar marinara sauce
- ✓ 1/2 cup feta cheese

Procedure:
1. Start by warming the oven to 370 degrees F.
2. In a large container, mix most of the ingredients aside from the cheese, oil, and marinara.
3. Mix well and create the meatballs.
4. Open the stove at medium settings and prepare a frying pan.
5. Start searing the meatballs.

6. Once done with the meatballs. Prepare an oven pan.
7. Pace the meatballs along with the marinara together.
8. Bake for 20 − 30 minutes.
9. Serve hot.

Yield: 16 meatballs

- Hot, Hot, Hot Salmon

Ingredients:
- ✓ 2 teaspoons chili powder
- ✓ 1 teaspoon ground cumin
- ✓ 1 teaspoon molasses
- ✓ 1/8 teaspoon salt
- ✓ 1/8 teaspoon black pepper
- ✓ 4 (4-ounce) salmon fillets
- ✓ Orange from half of an orange
- ✓ 2 tablespoons olive oil

Procedure:
1. Mix the pepper, sugar, chili powder, cumin, and salt.
2. Sprinkle the mixture onto the salmon.
3. Prepare a frying pan and set the stove to medium settings.
4. Add the salmon into the frying pan once hot. Cook for approximately 2 minutes.
5. Add the orange juice after 2 minutes on each face of the fillet.
6. Continue cooking for 3 more minutes.
7. Serve hot.

Yield: 4

- Taste of Mediterranean

Ingredients:
- ✓ 1 cup uncooked couscous
- ✓ 1 1/4 cups water
- ✓ 1 (16-ounce) can artichoke hearts
- ✓ 1/2 cup kalamata olives
- ✓ 1 (12-ounce) jar roasted red pepper
- ✓ 1/2 cup feta cheese
- ✓ 1 cup cherry tomatoes
- ✓ 1/2 small onion
- ✓ 1/4 teaspoon chopped oregano
- ✓ 1/4 teaspoon chopped fresh mint
- ✓ ½ teaspoon Pepper flakes
- ✓ 4 tablespoons extra virgin olive oil
- ✓ Lemon Juice from a Single Lemon
- ✓ A piece of Black Pepper

Procedure:
1. Start by boiling water and adding the couscous. Mix well.
2. Turn off the stove after mixing.
3. Cover the mixture and cool for 6 minutes.
4. In a separate container, combine the rest of the ingredients.
5. Place the mixture in the fridge for 17 minutes.
6. Mix the mixture with the couscous.
7. Serve chilled.

Yield: 4

Conclusion

Thank you again for getting this guide!

If you found this guide helpful, please take the time to share your thoughts and post a review. It would be greatly appreciated!

Thank you and good luck!

CPSIA information can be obtained
at www.ICGtesting.com
Printed in the USA
BVHW030227141122
651880BV00017B/488